I'm as surprised as you are that I'm writing this booklet.

When the coronavirus first emerged in China in January, I was researching American drug policy, working on a follow-up to *Tell Your Children,* my 2019 book on the mental health risks of cannabis.

But I couldn't stop reading about the virus – officially called SARS-COV-2. On conventional and social media, the news worsened by the day. Hospitals in the 10-million-person Chinese city of Wuhan were overrun. Videos on Twitter showed people dropping dead in the street and hospitals filled with body bags. Epidemiologists and scientists predicted the coronavirus would ravage other Chinese megacities.

In mid-February, the crisis seemed to pause. But by the end of the month, the coffins were stacking up in northern Italy, and the lockdowns beginning. Meanwhile, the United States reported its first deaths, at a nursing home in Seattle.

By early March I genuinely feared the United States might face an outbreak that would kill millions of Americans and potentially destabilize the nation. I loaded up on food for our family, bought the last N95 masks I could find at the local Wal-Mart, watched the stock market plunge.

Then, on Monday, March 16, Imperial College publicly released its now-infamous research report (https://www.imperial.ac.uk/media/imperial-college/medicine/sph/ide/gida-fellowships/Imperial-College-COVID19-NPI-modelling-16-03-2020.pdf) predicting coronavirus might kill a half-million Britons and two million Americans if governments didn't act immediately to close schools and businesses.

Worse, the report forecast 1.1 million Americans and 250,000 people in the United Kingdom could die even with months of efforts to reduce the damage. Only long-term "suppression" of society – possibly until a vaccine was invented – could lower those figures meaningfully, the researchers wrote.

The Imperial College researchers weren't just any academics. They worked directly with the World Health Organization. Their forecast terrified politicians across Europe and the United States and spurred what became a near-worldwide lockdown. Yet, ironically, the Imperial College report marked the beginning of my understanding of the realities of COVID-19. It planted the seeds of my skepticism about the lockdowns and our response to the coronavirus since.

Why?

When I read the report that Monday night, I noticed a chart on page 5 showing the likelihood of death in different age ranges. The chart showed coronavirus was more than 100 times as likely to kill people over 80 than under 50. Yes, 100 times. People under 30 were at very low risk.

The information stunned me. I knew coronavirus was more dangerous to older people, of course – but I assumed young people would also face serious risks. After all, any really deadly virus could hardly spare the young or middle-aged. A century ago, the Spanish flu killed children and young adults along with the elderly.

I found myself thinking of China. Not about what *had* happened in Wuhan, but about what *hadn't* happened everywhere else. Shanghai and Beijing and other huge cities had avoided catastrophe. In early

February, epidemiologists warned the Chinese lockdowns had come too late to matter. Instead, China was already tentatively reopening, restarting factories and dropping quarantines. If the virus was so deadly, how come the Chinese – who at that point had seen it more closely than anyone else – weren't more frightened?

I came back to the Page 5 chart again and again. I found myself asking two related questions: Why wasn't the media telling the truth about the huge difference in risk by age?

And was the coronavirus really as deadly as I and everyone else believed?

Nine days later, on March 25, the lead author of the Imperial College report, professor Neil Ferguson, testified about coronavirus to a committee of the British Parliament. Ferguson calls himself an epidemiologist, though he is not a physician and his doctorate is in theoretical physics. He was testifying remotely, since he had contracted the coronavirus a week before and was in a self-imposed home quarantine. (Later, a British newspaper would break the news that Ferguson had violated his isolation to have sex with a married woman he met on OKCupid; he was forced to resign in disgrace from a scientific committee advising the British government on the epidemic. But at the time his reputation was sterling and his previous forecasting mistakes – which are legion and in some cases comical – largely forgotten.)

Ferguson's testimony to the committee received no attention in the US. American media were focused on the emerging crisis in New York City. But British newspapers reported that Ferguson had dramatically changed his predictions. He now said his new best estimate was 20,000 Britons would die from the virus even with just weeks of quarantines.

Further, because the virus is far more dangerous to the elderly and people with severe health problems, more than half of those 20,000 people would probably have died in 2020 in any case, he said. (https://www.telegraph.co.uk/news/2020/03/25/two-thirds-patients-die-coronavirus-would-have-died-year-anyway/)

For the second time in just over a week, I found myself stunned. Instead of 500,000 British deaths, 20,000? Without months or years of lockdowns? In the absence of a vaccine or effective treatment? Had Ferguson just cut the Imperial College estimate by 96 percent (or 92 percent, if one used the 250,000-person death estimate)? What facts could have changed so much in just a few days? What did the change say about the accuracy of either the old or the new estimate?

And, again, why hadn't the New York Times and other American media outlets — after giving the earlier estimate so much attention — given equal prominence to the new number?

Investigative reporters have an old saw: *If your mother says she loves you, check it out.* In other words, question everything. But no one in the media seemed to be questioning anything. Instead, journalists were topping themselves with forecasts of doom. Molly Jong-Fast, an editor at the Daily Beast, told her 500,000 Twitter followers that as many as 7 percent of Americans — 23 million people — would die (https://twitter.com/mollyjongfast/status/1242508173627531269). The Times reporter Trip Gabriel predicted the United States was "expected" to need one million ventilators, the machines that breathe for people who can't on their own (https://twitter.com/tripgabriel/status/1242979481524076544?lang=en).

Gabriel's comment was absurd on its face. Ventilators are complex machines. Training physicians and respiratory therapists to use them takes years. Thus, even if we'd suddenly built a million ventilators, hospitals couldn't possibly have put people on them. If a million people at once were about to become so gravely ill that they needed ventilators, the apocalypse was truly nigh.

My instincts as an investigative reporter took over. I had been a New York Times reporter from 1999 until 2010, but I didn't work for the Times anymore. Even if I had been working for them, I doubted they would be interested in my efforts to challenge the narrative. They were among the leaders of what I had begun to think of as "Team Apocalypse," the media outlets that – for reasons I could not fully understand – seemed committed to painting as bleak a picture of the coronavirus as possible.

I had one outlet: Twitter. At the time I only had about 10,000 followers, but I was a verified account (in Twitter lingo, a blue-check), which gave me a bit of extra credibility. And I didn't have other options to ask questions in real time. The day after Ferguson's testimony, March 26, I raised questions about his revised estimate in a series of tweets.

For better or worse, people noticed. The most notable was Elon Musk, who besides being the founder of Tesla and SpaceX has a huge Twitter audience, with tens of millions of followers. Musk and others retweeted my primary tweet challenging Ferguson, and it was viewed almost 5 million times.

Suddenly I found myself as one of the few people with any journalistic standing challenging the apocalyptic reporting that dominated media outlets like the Times. Over the next few days, I pointed out on Twitter that a model from the University of Washington used to predict hospitalizations and intensive care needs was proving hugely wrong in its forecasts – even in New York, where the problems were worst.

Within a few days, "senior officials" in the White House had begun to notice the tweets and the questions they raised, according to New York Times reporter Maggie Haberman.
(https://twitter.com/maggienyt/status/1246805287627079681?lang=en)

Nonetheless, this view was less than popular, to say the least. Through late March and early April scorn and hate poured in, especially from my fellow media "blue-checks." People wished for me to die of coronavirus, which didn't really bother me, except when they said they hoped my family would too. The fear coming out of New York City, where so many members of the media lived, was palpable.

But as the days passed, the fact that the models were profoundly overestimating the number of people who would need to be hospitalized with SARS-COV-2 became self-evident. Despite repeated revisions, the model from the University of Washington continued to fail – not after months or even weeks, but on a daily basis.

In turn, the importance of that failure became increasingly obvious to me and a handful of other skeptics. What had happened in New York City in March was not generalizable to the rest of the United States. Hospitals outside New York were mostly empty and furloughing workers. Worse, in some cases they were *shutting down* because they had so few patients – a bizarre paradox in what was supposed to be the worst epidemic since the Spanish Flu a century before.
(https://www.alvareviewcourier.com/story/2020/04/10/regional/oklahoma-city-hospital-closed-amid-coronavirus-spread/62038.html)

Even in New York, the health-care system was never close to being overrun. Field hospitals built at a cost of tens of millions of dollars were dismantled; some had never seen a single patient. Navy hospital ships departed the harbor, searching in vain for new coronavirus hotspots. In late March, New York governor Andrew Cuomo had said the state might need 140,000 hospital beds and up to 40,000 ventilators. "Everybody's entitled to their own opinion, but I don't operate here on opinion. I operate on facts and on data and on numbers and on projections," Cuomo said.

https://www.syracuse.com/coronavirus/2020/03/cuomo-refutes-trump-insists-ny-needs-up-to-40000-ventilators-i-operate-on-facts.html

In the end, New York never had more than 4,000 coronavirus patients on ventilators – making Cuomo's facts and data and numbers and projections off by about tenfold.

By mid-April, it was obvious to me – and anyone who was paying attention – that the coronavirus epidemic simply was not going to be anywhere near as bad as the early predictions, and that the lockdowns were an extreme overreaction.

The failure of the models should have raised an even more crucial question: setting aside the massive economic and societal harms they'd caused, had the lockdowns even helped control the spread of the coronavirus at all?

But through April and May, major media outlets resolutely failed to ask that question. Instead, they focused nearly all their attention on COVID death counts, which rose slowly but steadily, eventually surpassing the total of 60,000 deaths initially estimated for the 2017-18 flu season.

Still, real information continued to drip out – often tucked away in scientific papers that went unnoticed, such as when a German research institute reported in mid-April that lockdowns had been broadly useless.

Yet – more than two months after they began – the lockdowns continue. Only Alaska has gone back to a pre-March normal. Even states like Georgia and Texas retain restrictions on restaurants and retailers and have not restarted their schools. Many other states, including giants like New York and Illinois, are repealing their rules slowly. In many cases they are requiring people to wear masks even in public and hinting that they will not allow schools to operate normally even in the fall.

So, yes, the coronavirus epidemic has largely ended as a medical crisis. But for now, the policies it has spawned remain educational, economic, and societal millstones. And the battles over issues such as mask-wearing, testing, contact tracing, and what to do if SARS-COV-2 regains momentum in the fall are burning hotter than ever.

Which is why I'm writing now.

I want to be clear my aims here are limited. I am not aiming here to provide a complete or even capsule history of SARS-COV-2, its initial spread in China in January, or the decisions that the United States and other countries made in February and March. For example, whether the virus emerged from of a Chinese biological research laboratory is a fascinating question. Eventually we may have a definitive answer. But for now anything I write would be speculation.

Nor will I spend time making specific judgments about coronavirus treatments. For example, I won't write about the various medicines now being tested for COVID, including hydroxychloroquine. Scientists and physicians are still examining those drugs in clinical trials. Until those trials are complete, even the doctors who use them can't be sure if they are working. For me to pretend I know what might work is worse than useless.

Eventually, I may write a longer book about SARS-COV-2 (I'll have lots of competition). If and when I do, I'll try to address the broader questions – though even a moderately comprehensive account may take years to research and write. The coronavirus, and the way we responded to it, will be grist for physicians and scientists and economists and historians and journalists for many years to come.

Instead of those broader topics, I want to focus here on crucial questions that I have tried to answer – or at least raise – in my Twitter feed in the last two months, including:

How lethal is SARS-COV-2? Is it more dangerous than the flu?

Who is most at risk?

How are SARS-COV-2 deaths coded? What questions does that coding policy raise?

What are the main ways in which the coronavirus has spread? How long has it been circulating?

How many people have already been infected?

Why did the key predictive models that policymakers used when they agreed to lockdowns prove so inaccurate?

Do lockdowns slow the spread?

What is the evidence for and against lockdowns, viewed on a public health basis, without regard to their economic, educational, and societal harms?

What about those other harms? How severe are they already, and how severe might they become?

What about the mental health risks of lockdowns?

Is requiring people to wear masks in public likely to slow the spread?

We can answer some of those questions more definitively than others, but after more than four months of frantic effort by scientists, they all have been at least partly unlocked. I will provide links to the papers and data I reference so you can judge whether the sourcing backs my answers.

I am committed to following the truth and offering the most honest answers, whatever they may be. I will not sugarcoat information, whether it is positive or negative.

For that reason, I've decided to dedicate the first chapter to discussing the number of potential deaths that the coronavirus in a worst-case scenario. As you'll see, the best estimate may be that 500,000 to 600,000 Americans might die in the next year or two.

That number is much lower than the initial Imperial College estimate, and roughly in the range of people whom smoking kills every year. Still, it is far higher than even a severe seasonal flu season – and may shock some people.

However, the estimate comes with three crucial caveats.

First, it assumes that we take NO efforts to protect the elderly, especially those in nursing homes, that we develop no medicines for coronavirus, and that physicians become no better at treating it. All three of those points are clearly wrong. States are moving to protect long-term care facilities (some, like Florida, did so early on). The antiviral medicine remdesivir has shown modest efficacy against COVID. And physicians have moved away from using ventilators aggressively, realizing that doing so can actually kill many coronavirus patients.

Second, it assumes that we will see a second wave of deaths: that the coronavirus, like the flu, will inevitably return this fall and winter. That view is the consensus among epidemiologists and scientists, and I won't challenge it (even though many epidemiologists have been badly wrong about COVID for the last three months). One counter-argument comes from Oxford University's Center for Evidence Based Medicine, which argued that "making absolute statements of certainty about 'second waves' is unwise, given the current substantial uncertainties and novelty of the evidence." (https://www.cebm.net/covid-19/covid-19-epidemic-waves/)

Third, and most importantly, the topline death figure does not account for the fact that the deaths will be heavily concentrated among the very old and sick. More than half would likely have died within weeks or months in any case, as Neil Ferguson said in his British testimony.

From any practical point of view, those deaths are unpreventable. Their timing is a function of the coronavirus, but their cause is underlying conditions such as cancer or heart disease or dementia. Meanwhile, children and young adults are at minimal risk from the virus.

Another way to look at deaths is to consider "life-years lost" – multiplying the number of deaths by the life expectancy of each person who has died. This measurement may seem cruel, but we all do it intuitively. Who would disagree that the death of a 10-year-old is harder to accept than, say, an 88-year-old? The child is only beginning her life; the man has already had his.

By the life-years standard, the coronavirus death toll appears more comparable to a single year of overdose deaths in the United States. About 70,000 people die from overdoses of opioids and other drugs every year, but they are on average far younger than those who die of coronavirus, so their overall life expectancy is similar.

Still, 600,000 deaths is a figure that can't be blinked away. As someone who has criticized lockdowns, I might seem to be hurting efforts to reopen by discussing it openly.

But it is precisely because the number appears so daunting that we must prepare for it – both practically, by monitoring hospitalizations closely and adding medical staff to hard-hit regions if necessary, and mentally, by refusing to panic again as we did in March if deaths begin to rise this fall. Going forward, we must remember the reason we locked down the United States and the rest of the world this spring was NOT to reduce coronavirus infections or deaths to zero. We have never pursued such a policy with any other respiratory virus, nor with viruses such as HIV, which until effective medicine existed killed nearly everyone who contracted it.

No, the reason we initially agreed to lockdowns was to "flatten the curve," which is a polite way of saying "to prevent coronavirus patients from collapsing our health-care system." But the system was never in danger of collapsing, lockdowns or no.

Now that that fact is clear, the lockdown rationale has shifted to the much more nebulous goal of reducing coronavirus deaths at any cost – as if deaths from COVID are the only kind of deaths or societal damage that matter.

The cost of this policy shift has been enormous. In less than three months, lockdowns have done incalculable damage. They need to be lifted as soon as possible. More importantly, we must agree that we will not restore them even if coronavirus deaths rise again in the fall and winter – unless hospitals face the real risk of collapse.

The changes we have already made to protect the most vulnerable, as well as individual efforts at social distancing – which are likely to continue even without government mandates – make a large wave of deaths less likely. But one is still possible. Thus we need to be prepared and realistic.

In general, I hope that what you read will both reassure you and help you pass information to friends and neighbors who may be unnecessarily frightened. A lot of what has happened over the last couple of months has been frustrating. But I've been lucky enough to have people tell me that my Twitter feed has helped make their lives a little more manageable. I hope this booklet can do the same. I believe reality will win, and that we will escape these lockdowns and return to normal as a society. But the road has already been longer and harder than I expected. The truth is our best weapon.

Onward.

(One final note – I have decided to release this booklet in sections; putting it together has already taken longer than I expected, and I want it to be a manageable length for an online read. I do plan to offer the combined sections in a single copy, both in paper and ebook.)

ONE

Maybe the most important questions of all:

How lethal is SARS-COV-2?

Whom does it kill?

Are the death counts accurate – and, if not, are they over- or understated?

Estimates for the lethality of the coronavirus have varied widely since January. Early Chinese data suggested the virus might have an "infection fatality rate" as high as 1.4 – 2 percent.

A death rate in that range could mean the coronavirus might kill more than 6 million Americans, although even under the worst-case scenarios some people would not be exposed, and others might have natural immunity that would prevent them from being infected at all.

As we have learned more about the virus, estimates of its lethality have fallen. Calculating fatality rates is complex, because despite all of our testing for COVID, we still don't know how many people have been infected.

Some people who are infected may have no or mild symptoms. Even those with more severe symptoms may resist going to the hospital, then recover on their own. We have a clear view of the top of the iceberg – the serious infections that require hospitalization – but at least in the early stages of the epidemic we have to guess at the mild, hidden infections.

But to calculate the true fatality rate, we need to know the true infection rate. If 10,000 people die out of 100,000 infections, that means the virus kills 10 percent of all the people it infects – making it very, very dangerous. But if 10,000 people die from 10 million infections, the death rate is actually 0.1 percent – similar to the flu.

Unfortunately, figuring out the real infection rate is very difficult. Probably the best way is through antibody tests, which measure how many people have already been infected and recovered – even if they never were hospitalized or even had symptoms. Studies in which many people in a city, state, or even country are tested at random to see if they are currently infected can also help. Believe it or not, so can tests of municipal sewage. (I'll say more about all this later, in the section on transmission rates and lockdowns.)

For now, the crucial point is this: randomized antibody tests from all over the world have repeatedly shown many more people have been infected with coronavirus than is revealed by tests for active infection. Many people who are infected with SARS-COV-2 don't even know it.

So the hidden part of the iceberg is huge. And in turn, scientists have repeatedly reduced their estimates for how dangerous the coronavirus might be.

The most important estimate came on May 20, when the Centers for Disease Control reported its best estimate was that the virus would kill 0.26 percent of people it infected, or about 1 in 400 people. (The virus would kill 0.4 percent of those who developed symptoms. But about one out of three people would have no symptoms at all, the CDC said.) (https://www.cdc.gov/coronavirus/2019-ncov/hcp/planning-scenarios.html#box.)

Similarly, a German study in April reported a fatality rate of 0.37 percent (https://www.technologyreview.com/2020/04/09/999015/blood-tests-show-15-of-people-are-now-immune-to-covid-19-in-one-town-in-germany/). A large study in April in Los Angeles predicted a death rate in the range of 0.15 to 0.3 percent.

Some estimates have been even lower. Others have been somewhat higher — especially in regions that experienced periods of severe stress on their health care systems. In New York City, for example, the death rates appear somewhat higher, possibly above 0.5 percent — though New York may be an outlier, both because it has counted deaths aggressively (more on this later) and because its hospitals seem to have used ventilators particularly aggressively.

Thus the CDC's estimate for deaths is probably the best place to begin. Using that figure along with several other papers and studies suggests the coronavirus has an infection fatality rate in the range of 0.15 percent to 0.4 percent.

In other words, SARS-COV-2 likely kills between 1 in 250 and 1 in 650 of the people whom it infects. Again, though, not everyone who is exposed will become infected. Some people do not contract the virus, perhaps because their T-cells — which help the immune system destroy invading viruses and bacteria — have already been primed by exposure to other coronaviruses. [Several other coronaviruses exist; the most common versions usually cause minor colds in the people they infect.] An early May paper in the journal Cell suggests that as many as 60 percent of people may have some preexisting immune response, though not all will necessarily be immune. (https://www.cell.com/cell/pdf/S0092-8674(20)30610-3.pdf).

The experience of outbreaks on large ships such as aircraft carriers and cruise liners also show that some people do not become infected. The best estimates are that the virus probably can infect somewhere between 50 to 70 percent of people. For example, on one French aircraft carrier, 60 percent of sailors were infected (none died and only two out of 1,074 infected sailors required intensive care).
https://www.navalnews.com/naval-news/2020/05/covid-19-aboard-french-aircraft-carrier-98-of-the-crew-now-cured/

Thus – in a worst-case scenario – if we took no steps to mitigate its spread or protect vulnerable people, a completely unchecked coronavirus might kill between 0.075 and 0.28 percent of the United States population – between 1 in 360 and 1 in 1,300 Americans.

This is **higher** than the seasonal flu in most years. Influenza is usually said to have a fatality rate among symptomatic cases of 1 in 1,000 and an overall fatality rate of around 1 in 2,000. However, influenza mutates rapidly, and its dangerousness varies year by year. The coronavirus appears far less dangerous than the Spanish flu a century ago, which was commonly said to kill 1 in 50 of the people it infected.

It appears more comparable in terms of overall mortality to the influenza epidemics of 1957 and 1968, or the British flu epidemics of the late 1990s. (Of course, the United States and United Kingdom did not only not shut down for any of those epidemics, they received little attention outside the health-care system.)

Viewed another way: On a per-person basis, the coronavirus risk is relatively small. But the United States is a big country, so on a population level the overall potential fatality numbers are eye-catching. They represent a worst-case death toll of 250,000 to 900,000 Americans. The Centers for Disease Control's estimate translates into a range of just over a half-million total coronavirus deaths, for example.

The topline coronavirus death toll is important. But arguably even more important questions are who is dying – and how long those people might have lived if the coronavirus had not killed them.

Unfortunately, those have received far less media attention, though the answers could not be clearer. Coronavirus overwhelmingly targets the very old and sick. And when they die many of those people have at most months to live.

Just how old? The median age of people killed by the coronavirus is roughly 80 to 82 worldwide. (Median represents the halfway point – half of all people are older and half younger.)

A few examples: as of May 28, the median age of the 32,000 Italians killed by COVID-19 was 81. More than 13,000 were over 80. Another 5,400 were over 90. (https://www.epicentro.iss.it/en/coronavirus/bollettino/Report-COVID-2019_28_may_2020.pdf)

In England and Wales, as of May 15, about 17,000 of the 41,000 coronavirus deaths occurred in people over 85. Another 13,000 occurred in people between 75 and 84.

(https://www.ons.gov.uk/peoplepopulationandcommunity/healthandsocialcare/conditionsanddiseases/articles/coronaviruscovid19roundup/2020-03-26)

In New York, as of May 28, almost 40 percent of the 23,700 reported deaths occurred in people over 80. (https://covid19tracker.health.ny.gov/views/NYS-COVID19-Tracker/NYSDOHCOVID-19Tracker-Fatalities?%3Aembed=yes&%3Atoolbar=no&%3Atabs=n)

In Minnesota, the median age of the 1,000 COVID deaths is almost 84. More people over 100 have died than under 50. (https://www.health.state.mn.us/diseases/coronavirus/stats/covidweekly22.pdf)

The pattern is the same everywhere. Extremely elderly people are far more likely to die of SARS-COV-2 than anyone else. That is especially true for those living in nursing homes and assisted living facilities. Those people account for about 40 to 50 percent of all deaths from COVID in the United States. A figure of 43 percent has been widely used. It probably understates the real total because in some states, including New York, nursing home residents who die in hospitals are counted as hospital deaths. (https://www.forbes.com/sites/theapothecary/2020/05/26/nursing-homes-assisted-living-facilities-0-6-of-the-u-s-population-43-of-u-s-covid-19-deaths/#1a759cff74cd)

The flip side of the risk to the elderly is that younger adults and especially teenagers and children are at extremely low risk from SARS-COV-2. In Italy, a total of 17 people under 30 have died of the coronavirus. In the United Kingdom, four people under 15 have died. In New York, 14 under 20 and 102 under 30.

Worldwide, it is almost certain that more people **over the age of 100** than **under 30** have died of SARS-COV-2. Many more children die of influenza than coronavirus; in the 2019-20 flu season, the Centers for Disease Control received about 180 reports of pediatric flu deaths. It has received 19 reports of coronavirus deaths in children under 15 so far.

This profound difference in risk by age has been obvious at least since mid-March, as the Imperial College report showed. It may only have grown since then, in part because misguided government policies in many states and some European countries needlessly exposed many nursing home residents to the coronavirus.

But most people have no idea how large the gap might be, because public health authorities and lawmakers have rarely discussed it honestly. To hide the reality, authorities often refer to the age distribution of coronavirus "cases." For example, Dr. Judith Malmgren, a Washington state epidemiologist, said on May 30 (!), "We need to make it clear that it's an equal opportunity disease." She cited the growth in "cases" in people under 40.

https://www.king5.com/article/news/health/coronavirus/seattle-epidemiologist-concerned-about-spike-of-coronavirus-in-those-under-40/281-1845991d-a1f0-4530-932a-cb29ae06be7f)

But a "case" of coronavirus refers only to a positive test result showing someone has been infected. It does not mean that a person will become sick – much less that he or she will be hospitalized, need intensive care, or die. Thus discussing the age distribution of infections, while technically not untruthful, is extremely misleading.

Major media outlets like the Times and Washington Post have gone the other way, focusing enormous attention on the literal handful of cases where children or young adults may have died from coronavirus. On Twitter, reporters go further. A Washington Post reporter tweeted on May 28, "Who among us today will be dead by next month? Your cashier at the grocery store? Your best friend? Your child?"
https://twitter.com/kemettler/status/1266000325942685697

Worst of all, as it has become obvious that active infections are generally harmless to kids or young adults, media outlets and public health authorities have highlighted the potential for very rare post-infection inflammatory and immune syndromes that cause heart damage or even kill children. Other infections are also known to cause such syndromes, so the fact that SARS-COV-2 might should not be shocking. Yet the media has treated the possibility as unprecedented rather than putting it in context.

As a father, I understand why parents might be worried. But from everything we have learned in the last few months, the coronavirus is less dangerous to children than the flu, much less other common threats to kids including car accidents, drownings – and child abuse. (I'll discuss this issue more in a later booklet when in the section on schools and school reopenings.)

The shockingly wide age differential of coronavirus deaths has another major consequence – it makes properly counting and attributing deaths to the virus much more difficult.

The United States and other countries count coronavirus deaths extremely aggressively. On March 24, the Centers for Disease Control issued new guidelines for reporting coronavirus deaths, saying explicitly that "the rules for coding and selection of the underlying cause of death are expected to result in COVID19 (sic) being the underlying cause more often than not." Notably, the CDC did not require a positive coronavirus test for physicians, coroners, or health departments to find that the virus had caused the death.

"Should 'COVID-19' be reported on the death certificate only with a confirmed test? [No], COVID-19 should be reported on the death certificate for all decedents where the disease caused or **is assumed to have caused or contributed to death.** [Emphasis added.]"

https://www.cdc.gov/nchs/data/nvss/coronavirus/Alert-2-New-ICD-code-introduced-for-COVID-19-deaths.pdf

Many states assume that anyone with a positive coronavirus test has died from the disease, no matter what their actual cause of death. As the director of the Illinois Department of Public Health explained in April, "If you were in hospice and had already been given a few weeks to live, and then you were also found to have COVID, that would be counted as a COVID death. It means technically even if you died of a clear alternate cause, but you had COVID at the same time, it's still listed as a COVID death."

https://week.com/2020/04/20/idph-director-explains-how-covid-deaths-are-classified/

The anomalies extend past deaths of hospice patients. For example, Washington state reported on May 21 it had included five people who had died of gunshots in its total of roughly 1,000 coronavirus deaths. (https://www.clarkcountytoday.com/news/washington-department-of-health-clarifies-covid-19-death-numbers/)

Further, to make sure they don't miss any potential cases, some states match databases of deaths of people who have died with those who had positive coronavirus test results – and add anyone with a positive test result to their counts, even if there was no initial finding that coronavirus caused the death. (https://jtv.tv/michigan-reports-263-coronavirus-cases-today-state-total-now-56884/)

Just how many "gunshot wound"-type deaths are in the COVID counts? We cannot be sure, because most states have not disclosed them.

Colorado is an exception. It reports both "deaths among people with COVID-19" and "deaths from people who died from COVID-19."

As of June 2, Colorado reported 1,474 "deaths among cases" but 1,228 "deaths due to COVID-19," a gap of roughly 17 percent.
https://covid19.colorado.gov/data/case-data

(The widely watched "worldometers.info" Website uses the higher figure; also, 804 of the "deaths among cases" occurred in people over 80, while 18 occurred in people under 40.) If the same gap applies nationally, almost 20,000 of the deaths that have been attributed to the coronavirus have at most a tenuous connection to it.

I don't mean to imply here that COVID-19 is not lethal or that most deaths listed as COVID-19 in the United States are not in some way related to the virus. The bubble of deaths in New York City in March and April is inarguable. Roughly 32,000 people died in the city over an eight-week period, about four times as many as in a normal spring. About 14,000 of those deaths were definitely COVID-related and another 5,000 were probably COVID-related.
https://www.cdc.gov/mmwr/volumes/69/wr/mm6919e5.htm

But major media outlets have repeatedly tried to make the case that somehow the United States has sharply undercounted coronavirus deaths. The fact that a significant fraction of deaths already listed as caused coronavirus are in fact "deaths among cases" strongly suggests otherwise.

An even more serious and ultimately insoluble problem in the count comes not from the coding of some deaths that are clearly unrelated to the virus as COVID-related, but because the vast majority of people who die after becoming infected with coronavirus are old and unwell.

In these cases, the distinction between dying WITH coronavirus as opposed to FROM coronavirus can be nearly impossible to make.

Determining the cause of death can be a messy process. Coroners and health authorities must frequently balance an underlying illness with the event that specifically killed someone. Sometimes doing so is easy. An apparently healthy 55-year-old man who dies of a heart attack caused by a clot in his artery has died of coronary artery disease. But what if the man has diabetes, which can cause heart problems? Should the death be attributed to diabetes or heart disease?

Or what if man drinks too much, drives his car into a tree, and bleeds to death before he can be rescued? His immediate cause of death is the hemorrhage. The accident caused the hemorrhage. But most people would agree the real cause of death in this case is alcohol abuse.

In those examples, at least, cause and effect is clear. But for contagious illnesses that mainly kill people already near death from serious underlying conditions, sorting out the "real" cause of death may be impossible.

A 2012 Canadian Broadcasting Corporation article on estimates for flu deaths highlighted this issue. Canada reports up to 8,000 deaths from influenza every year, the equivalent of more than 70,000 in the United States. But as the article noted, "Death can be complicated. If someone already extremely fragile with heart or lung disease is tipped over the edge with a flu infection, is that a flu death, or a heart death or a lung death? Which database gets to claim it?"
https://www.cbc.ca/news/health/flu-deaths-reality-check-1.1127442

Coronavirus targets people at the end of their lives even more aggressively than the flu, so the issue is even more serious. Beside Neil Ferguson's testimony in March, the fact that so many coronavirus deaths occur in nursing home patients is strong evidence that many victims had only weeks or months to live. By the time they come to nursing homes, most people are very frail. A 2010 study in the Journal of the American Geriatrics Society found that half of all people admitted to nursing homes died within five months of admission (though the average length of stay was longer, because a fraction of residents lived several years after admission).

https://onlinelibrary.wiley.com/doi/abs/10.1111/j.1532-5415.2010.03005.x

Thus, over the course of a year or two, the coronavirus is likely to have little if any impact on the overall number of Americans who die, **even if the worst-case estimates for overall mortality are correct.** If 600,000 people die of coronavirus by the time everyone is exposed to it, but two-thirds of them would have died anyway from other illnesses, the "excess" mortality from coronavirus – people who would would not have died during that period – would be 200,000 people.

But almost 6 million people die every two years in the United States. Thus 200,000 deaths would represent an increase in mortality of a little over 3 percent for the entire nation. Two hundred thousand extra deaths also equals about the same number of people who die from alcohol abuse over a two-year period, or from overdoses over a three-year-period.

Yes, coronavirus kills.

It's not alone.

Made in the USA
Monee, IL
15 June 2020

33177038R00016